All You Can Eat Free Foods

Vegetables, Meats, Seafood and Beverages Grocery List

Paula C. Henderson

DEDICATION

To all those who went hungry on a diet but didn't need to!
.

CONTENTS

Published Works By Paula C. Henderson

How I Got Free Stuff To Sell Online And Quit My Job
ASIN Kindle B01KGP8FZU http://amzn.to/2kP8wRF
ISBN Paperback 1542880653 http://amzn.to/2lpmnBu

Dictionary of Cooking Terms for the Beginner Cook
ASIN Kindle: B01L88R4EM http://amzn.to/2kP3epv

Tips For Your Weight Loss Success
ASIN Kindle B01LYVVC1S http://amzn.to/2kDLmNc
ISBN Paperback 1539143457 http://amzn.to/2kY3mVV

All You Can Eat Free Foods
Kindle edition: http://amzn.to/2kDQIYN
Paperback ISBN: **1543155278**

Lettuce Amaze You
Kindle ASIN: B01N1P34BK http://amzn.to/2lTNXEr
Paperback ISBN: 1540874931 http://amzn.to/2kPgLND

What's Left To Eat Grocery List
Kindle ASIN: B01N7F2NQB http://amzn.to/2kDZfef

A Gluten and Dairy Free, Grain Free, Soy Free, and Nightshade Free
Grocery List: This is **"What's Left To Eat"**
Paperback ISBN: 1542622727 http://amzn.to/2kPafGH

1 FREE FOODS

We have all heard of free foods. Those foods that have little or no fat content and little or no carbs but offer great nutritional value. The most commonly known is celery. None exist in the fruit group because all fruits have sugar content and sugar, even natural sugars, are carbs.

Below you will find a list of more than 80 foods that are 5 Points Diet Plan friendly. Healthy, low carb, naturally low in sugar, low fat, and low in sodium foods. There is no reason these should not be a part of anyone's regular diet. This list is also dairy free, gluten free, soy free, grain free and nightshade free.

Certainly a great list to refer to if you want to lose a few pounds or just watch your calorie intake for a day or two. There is an unlimited possibility of salad variations you could create just using this list of vegetables. Make some great stir fry's or a vegetable soup. How about grilled veggies? Or puree some cauliflower with chicken broth and garlic? A creamy asparagus, cauliflower, or broccoli soup that is dairy free and delicious?

2 VEGETABLES

- Artichokes –

  - Artichokes are an excellent substitute if you are avoiding tomatoes.

- Arugula

- Asparagus

  - Fresh asparagus best prep?

    Toss with oil, salt and pepper and bake in the oven until tender or you can grill them.

    It is also very easy to make a quick cream of asparagus soup for well, soup or you can use it as a sauce. Cooked asparagus (fresh, frozen or canned is fine) in the blender, add one cup chicken broth, salt and pepper. Blend until smooth adding more broth until it is the consistency you like. Sauté garlic in a saucepan, add the soup, heat through after blending.

- Basil

  - Great plant to have in your home. Snip it as needed and let it grow right back! Make pesto as a substitute for tomato sauce on pizza and on pasta and other Italian dishes. Basic pesto is merely basil or spinach leaves, garlic cloves (more than usual), a squirt of lime juice, oil, salt and pepper. Some like to add parmesan cheese and/or pine nuts.

- Bibb Lettuce:

  - great for lettuce cups. Use in place of taco shells, sandwich bread and buns to lower your carb intake.

- Bok Choy - Great for stir fry!

- Broccoli

  - Cruciferous so avoid raw if you are living with hypothyroidism, fine consume cooked.

    Make cream of broccoli soup using the same method as the asparagus soup. This needs to be blended and blended. It will get nice and creamy smooth but you will feel like you are blending it to death. But it works and that is all that matters in the end. A wonderful soup on a cold day.

- Brussel Sprouts

  - cruciferous so avoid raw, always consume cooked if you have been diagnosed with hypothyroidism

- Cabbage

  o cruciferous (see broccoli) Cabbage is also a rich source of vitamin K. A good thing for most of us but if you take blood thinners you should be aware of any food with a significant amount of Vitamin K.

  o Cabbage is an excellent source of fiber. So if you find yourself constipated this may be just the thing. Saute some cabbage with onion and ground beef for a quick meal. Chop cabbage thinly, toss with mayo and enjoy fish tacos for supper! Sauerkraut is cabbage! So enjoy some sauerkraut.

  o Cabbage is very low carb but full of Vitamin C so it is good for your immune system, hair, eyes, skin and nails.

  o Look up some recipes for a nice cabbage soup.

  o For a quick weeknight recipe: sauté cabbage and onion with hamburger, add some frozen green peas, add just a squirt of yellow mustard, salt and pepper.

- Carrots

  o This is a borderline food as far as if it is a high carb food or not. You can easily eat a normal portion of carrots daily and it should not be a problem. Highly nutritious too!

  I enjoy Carrot Puree for breakfast most mornings. Drained canned carrots, or cooked fresh carrots (reserve the liquid). Allow to cool if you just boiled (I generally will boil the night before and blend next morning). Blend with part of the liquid and add more liquid to the consistency of cream of wheat. Heat through. Add honey, cinnamon, nutmeg and a little real butter. If you want a milder carrot taste, add a cooked apple (just boil with fresh carrots). When preparing this leave the peels on! And blend all together. Pears are very nice too in this dish.

- Cauliflower

  o Cruciferous so avoid raw, always consume cooked. Fresh or frozen this is a versatile vegetable.

  For a quick side put cooked cauliflower, or frozen right out of the bag, and blend in the blender with chicken broth (that you hopefully made from preparing chicken) and whatever seasonings you like for a mashed cauliflower. Be sure to add the liquid a tiny bit at a time to get the right consistency. Heat through before serving.

  Another prep that is trending right now is to cut a whole, raw cauliflower head lengthwise into 3 or 4 slices.

Drizzle generously with oil, salt and pepper. Bake until tender and brown. Or, you could put it on the grill. A squirt of lime or lemon juice before servings is especially good. A cauliflower steak is the perfect place for cilantro or parsley salad:

Chop fresh cilantro or parsley, toss with oil, salt and pepper and a squirt of apple cider vinegar (to taste). Let the salad sit for at least an hour before serving. Especially good spread atop a cauliflower steak or a ribeye.

- Celery, celery leaves and celery root

   o A stalk of celery will stay fresh a lot longer if you wrap it tightly in aluminum foil. Since I avoid nightshades I use celery anywhere I would have used green bell pepper. I rarely eat just a stalk of celery but I do keep it on hand for dicing into salads, soups and sauces. If you like stuffed celery sticks try mixing an avocado with a little horseradish and stuff some celery sticks with that for those looking for something with a kick.

   If you are not a big fan of celery try this for the best possible tasting celery: Wash and cut into edible celery sticks. Place in a glass bowl that has a lid. Like Rubbermaid or Pyrex storage bowls with the red lids. Cover with water and the lid! Refrigerate overnight (at least 6 hours before serving). This improves the look, texture and taste of your celery.

- Chives -

- Cilantro

  o I use this for almost everything so I grow my own. You have to grow a lot if you use a lot but it's a pretty plant.

  I toss in salads, put in lettuce cups, tortilla wraps, salsa, guacamole, soups, dips and salad dressings, sauces, I sprinkle on top of prepared foods too.

  Try this quick cilantro salad to add to a salad, or enjoy on top meats and vegetable dishes:

  Chop fresh cilantro, toss with oil, salt, pepper, apple cider vinegar to taste. Add chopped or diced onion (optional). Prepare this about an hour before serving. (You could also use parsley)

- Collard Greens

  o Garlicky sautéed collards are great under roasted meats. Or chop and add to soups. For more in depth flavor I like to sauté mine with some chicken broth and garlic. Let the broth cook out over medium heat.

- Cucumbers

  o Very hydrating. Great base for making a quick salad dressing or a dip. Sliced cucumber that has been peeled is especially nice to put out when you are serving a heavy meal like meatloaf or a spicy meal. I always leave the peel on when I am blending them for a dressing or dip.

- Dandelion

- Dill -

- Endive -

- Fennel –

- Fiddlehead

- Frisee

- Garlic –

    o I buy fresh garlic bulbs, place in freezer bag and keep in freezer.

- Ginger Root

    o Wash and place in freezer bag. Easily slices or grates for each use and then return to freezer.

- Green Beans

    o Toss fresh or frozen whole green beans with oil, salt and pepper and sauté in a little garlic and chicken stock' or bake until tender. Best if they turn a golden brown.

- Herbs

    o Grow fresh herbs yourself or buy fresh in produce or dried in the aisles. These are also becoming more readily available in the freezer section.

- Horseradish Root

- Iceberg Lettuce

- Kale

  o cruciferous so avoid raw, always consume cooked

- Leeks -

- Lemon Grass -

- Lettuce:

  o all lettuce! Arugula, iceberg, romaine, bib, leaf, radicchio, watercress. Any lettuce. -

- Mushrooms: All mushrooms

  o Exception: avoid mushrooms if you have been diagnosed with candida or have recurring yeast infections.

- Mustard Greens - , cruciferous so avoid raw, always consume cooked. Note: steamed or sautéed mustard and collard greens are great for lowering cholesterol.

- Okra

  o Have you tried tossing whole okra with oil, salt and pepper and baking until golden brown? Hit it with the broiler before taking out to brown if needed. Turn half way through cooking.

- Olives

- Onions: all onions –

- Parsley

  - All parsley does not taste like the other. So try different kinds. Parsley is a healthy addition to many meals that might otherwise go without a vegetable!

- Radicchio

- Radishes

  - Recipe Bonus: Frozen peas (rinse in warm water) tossed with sliced radishes, oil, salt, pepper and apple cider vinegar or lime juice. Serve cold. Makes a nice side dish or toss with fresh spinach or romaine. Also good with a honey mustard dressing: mix equal parts yellow mustard with honey. Adjust to taste.

- Rhubarb – if the recipe you are using includes only free foods than rhubarb is also a free food. The problem comes in when we use rhubarb in a traditionally common way and add too much sugar to our diets.

- Romaine Lettuce

- Seasonings and spices

- Sage -

- Snow Peas

- Sugar Peas

- Snap Peas –

- Spaghetti Squash –

  o Most recipes call for baking this in the oven after having to cut it in half, raw. Personally I find that terribly difficult. I boil mine and then cut it in half after it has cooked. Boil it whole. You'll know it's done when a knife slides into the rind easily. Allow it to cool before cutting in half. Use an ice cream scoop to easily remove the seeds and a fork to remove the flesh.

- Spinach

  o Wonderful plant to have in your home. Snip it as needed and let it grow right back! Make pesto as a substitute for tomato sauce on pizza, on pasta and other Italian dishes.

- Swiss Chard -

- Turnip Greens

- Watercress

- Yellow Squash –

- Zucchini

  o Best prep tip is to cut lengthwise. Rub all over in oil, salt and pepper and put it on the grill until turning brown and tender. You must try this at least once. So good!

A note about cruciferous vegetables: some people, one example are those of us with hypothyroidism, should not eat raw cruciferous vegetables. They are perfectly fine, and very healthy. Just make sure you cook them before consumption. Cruciferous vegetables include: kale, broccoli, cabbage, and cauliflower. If you find even cooked cruciferous bothers you simply avoid them. We are all unique; if you find one or all of them cause you problems do not eat them. They are not necessary for overall good health as there are plenty of other vegetables to choose from.

3 PANTRY (AISLES)

- Asparagus

  - Canned. Drain a can of asparagus, using your can as a measuring cup, add a can of chicken stock. Blend until smooth. In a sauté pan heat some oil, sauté some garlic, add the broth and asparagus. Add salt and pepper to taste. If you want a creamy thicker Cream of Asparagus soup, remove a ladle of soup to a bowl. Add two tablespoons of arrowroot or gluten free flour and stir till smooth. Bring soup in saucepan to a light boil and add the slurry slowly while stirring constantly. You could also add shredded chicken you boiled and pulled from the bone for a heartier evening meal.

- Anchovies

- Bamboo Shoots

- Broth/Stock: Low Sodium!!

  o Homemade is your best bet. Chicken, beef, vegetable, bone, or mushroom broth. Best to make yourself and don't add anything but the meat or mushrooms. Bone-in meats make the best broth. Every few weeks I will buy a large bag of chicken breasts and/or chicken thighs and when on sale a whole chicken. Boil on med-low heat covered in plain water. Keep at a low boil. Don't add anything but the chicken.

  o When the chicken is done (close to falling off the bone) remove and allow to cool. The chicken can be left in whole pieces (freeze for a quick sandwich or to heat and put under a nice sauce), for a chicken sandwich or use a fork and pull apart for chicken tacos, lettuce cups, chicken salad, pulled chicken sandwiches, or for your chicken vegetable soup that I know you are going to make using that great broth you just made!

  o The Broth: First allow to cool, uncovered on the counter. Then cover and set in frig overnight. This allows the fat to separate from the broth. Remove the fat from the top and freeze the pure low fat, low sodium broth. I like to freeze in ice cube trays, then transfer to freezer bags to use as needed. I keep some in the refrigerator in a jar that I have labeled for immediate use during the week. When you make it yourself you know you have not added any sodium and it really does taste better. If you try it let me know!

- Canned Tuna in Water:

  - Keep in mind that half a can is one serving according to a 5 ounce can of tuna in water. According to the nutritional label half a can, or one serving has 170 mg of sodium. So depending on your sodium needs or need to avoid will decide if this can be a free food for you or not. If you are going to use it as a 'free food' please not only drain the tuna but rinse it prior to consumption. It also helps to pair it with other foods that are virtually sodium free.

- Capers

- Cooking Spray (nonstick)

- Green Beans

  - canned. Be sure the ingredients are limited to green beans, water, and salt. For that matter, any vegetable listed in the Vegetable list above is a free food even from a can or the frozen foods department. Just check the ingredient list. Water, salt and broth are the only other ingredients that are okay. Not any type of starch, spices or additives or unfamiliar items. If it isn't on this list you do not want it.

- Mushrooms

- Olives

- Sauerkraut

- Sesame Oil

- Vinegar:

    o all kinds of vinegar with the exception of malt vinegar.

- Water Chestnuts

- Yellow mustard

4 REFRIGERATED SECTION

- Eggs

- Unsweetened Original Almond Milk

5 PRODUCE DEPARTMENT

- All the vegetables on the list above.

- Lemons and limes (juice and their zest) If you are vulnerable to Restless Leg Syndrome or an Overactive Bladder please avoid all citrus including lemons and limes.

6 FROZEN FOODS

FROZEN FOODS

- All vegetables listed in the vegetables list

7 MEAT AND SEAFOOD

- o As long as you are buying whole, fresh, meats and seafood (no pre-cooked or seasoned) and you are preparing it only with other products on this list, meat and seafood is a free food. Be sure to keep it a free food by preparing it with only other ingredients on this list. Examples of whole, fresh meats and seafood choices:

- o Poultry: Turkey, ground turkey, Chicken breasts, hen, fryer, wings and thighs. Find these in the meat department, not the frozen foods where the chicken is precooked and seasoned.

- o Beef: ground beef, unseasoned, steak, roast, ribs. TIP: you can make a meatloaf without adding flour, breadcrumbs or crackers as a binder. Make the meatloaf with never before frozen hamburger. Make sure it is 90% lean or higher. Add seasonings and egg (optional) only. Do not add ketchup as it is a nightshade and you will notice ketchup is not on this list. Ketchup is also a highly processed food.

- o Pork: ground pork in lieu of breakfast sausage or Italian sausage. Instead add seasoning yourself at home. You do not want to consume cured, pre-cooked meats. Ribs, roast, pork chops.

- o Seafood: salmon filets, cod, tilapia, shrimp, tuna, scallops, catfish, perch, white fish.

    Suggested preparation: poaching, grilling, baking, and steaming. Use water, broth, seasonings, herbs, other vegetables to flavor the meat; not oils.

8 BEVERAGES

- o Water
- o Sparkling Water; unflavored

  (you can use fresh lime or cucumber)
- o Unsweetened Original Almond Milk
- o Unsweetened Tea

9 MENU IDEAS

Please remember to limit the foods used to prepare your meats to the foods on this list. That, of course, means no dusting in flour. While cooking oil is not listed here as an "All You Can Eat Free Food" it is a food you can use sparingly in order to prepare your foods. For the best tasting, simply prepared whole meats such as chicken breasts, steak, pork chops, and seafood I suggest rubbing with a minimal amount of oil, salt and pepper and then bake or Sear your meat or seafood on both sides in a skillet, add broth of your choice; just enough to cover the bottom of the skillet not cover the meat, and simmer until your broth has cooked out. This is a great way to impart some flavor into your dish. You can also add seasonings to your broth. Or, of course, there is the crock pot which is great for roasts and more.

Let's start with the obvious: **Salads**!

Any combination of the vegetables on this list constitutes a salad. And keep it interesting; not all salads have to be lettuce with toppings and dressing. Mix it up!

Try a cup of chopped cilantro, diced onion, and shredded carrot. Toss with oil, salt, pepper and a squirt of apple cider vinegar. Best when allowed to sit at least an hour before serving.

Make a salad of chopped cucumber, purple onion, black or Kalamata olives with fresh spinach leaves; toss with oil, salt and pepper and Italian seasoning.

Here is an out of the ordinary lettuce salad: Cut your lettuce into thin slices instead of chunks. Add frozen peas that have been rinsed in warm water to thaw. Also add shredded carrot and some thin slices of celery as well as thinly sliced radishes. Toss with oil, vinegar (or lime juice), garlic, salt and pepper.

Roasted Vegetables: Toss with oil, salt and pepper. Grill or bake until golden brown and tender. Best vegetable choices: mushrooms, zucchini, carrots, onions, artichokes, squash, cauliflower, asparagus and green beans. Romaine hearts, leeks, Brussel sprouts, whole okra.

Soup: An easy go-to comforting meal. Place your vegetables of choice in the crock pot with some broth or stock, meat if you like and let it do the cooking for you! Don't forget the bay leaf.

Try some **one skillet dinners** like ground beef, pork or turkey and add a can of drained green beans. Sounds boring, taste great! Add olives, onions, and Italian seasonings for a flavor twist. What about chicken thighs browned in the skillet and then add onions, a can of artichokes and asparagus tips?

Pureed Vegetables: Pureed Cauliflower. Tip, use chicken broth instead of water to add flavor. Do you like asparagus? Cream of Asparagus soup? Puree cooked asparagus with chicken broth. Transfer to saucepan and add garlic, salt and pepper. Heat through. If your creamy soup seems like it needs something to brighten it up try a squirt of apple cider vinegar. Of course you could also use broccoli in place of the asparagus, or cauliflower.

Looking for more ideas? Join our 5 Points Diet Plan group on facebook! #5ptsfreediet

ABOUT THE AUTHOR

Paula C. Henderson is a Nutritionist, Weight Loss Counselor and Author who makes her home in Las Vegas, Nevada. Creator of the 5pts Free Diet which promotes easing your symptoms from auto-immune, inflammation, depression, insomnia, obesity, hypothyroid, menopause, arthritis and more through diet and a healthy lifestyle.

Paula grew up in Illinois and then moved to Ohio where, as a single mother, raised her daughter.

Becoming a certified weight loss counselor started an interest in healthy food choices and a healthy lifestyle that continues today. Taking care of one's self is even more important when facing daily challenges. Through the years Paula has continued her education as a Nutritionist and health care advocate.

Paula has written several books on diet and nutrition. By following Paula you will get a notification as she releases each new book.

Find all of her books on Amazon.

amazon.com/author/paulachenderson

www.ingramcontent.com/pod-product-compliance
Lightning Source LLC
Chambersburg PA
CBHW071322280526
45788CB00004B/1993